THE NO COMPROMISE BLACK SKIN CARE GUIDE

THE TRUTH ABOUT CARING FOR DARKER SKIN

C. R COOPER: THE SKIN THEOLOGIAN

Let's connect either on instagram
IG: @theskintheologian (or) at
www.skintheologian.com

© **Copyright Charmaine Cooper 2021 - All rights reserved.**

The content contained within this book may not be reproduced, duplicated or transmitted without direct written permission from the author or the publisher.

Under no circumstances will any blame or legal responsibility be held against the publisher, or author, for any damages, reparation, or monetary loss due to the information contained within this book. Either directly or indirectly. You are responsible for your own choices, actions, and results.

Legal Notice:

This book is copyright protected. This book is only for personal use. You cannot amend, distribute, sell, use, quote or paraphrase any part, or the content within this book, without the consent of the author or publisher.

Disclaimer Notice:

Please note the information contained within this document is for educational and entertainment purposes only. All effort has been executed to present accurate, up to date, and reliable, complete information. No warranties of any kind are declared or implied. Readers acknowledge that the author is not engaging in the rendering of legal, financial, medical or professional advice. The content within this book has been derived from various sources. Please consult a licensed professional before attempting any techniques outlined in this book.

By reading this document, the reader agrees that under no circumstances is the author responsible for any losses, direct or indirect, which are incurred as a result of the use of the information contained within this document, including, but not limited to, — errors, omissions, or inaccuracies.

CONTENTS

Introduction	9
Who am I?	15
1. Skin Theology	17
2. The Skin Pro's Perspective	36
3. More Than Skin Deep	61
4. Primary and Common Concerns with Black Skin	80
5. Let's Level-Up on Ingredients	95
6. Treatment Solutions	112
7. The Skin Theologian's 10 Commandments for Black Skin	120
Conclusion	123
Skin color in dermatology textbooks: An updated evaluation and analysis	127

This resource is dedicated to every skin professional, new or well seasoned, and to every skin enthusiastic consumer who ever struggled with confidently treating black skin.

I got you.

SPECIAL SKIN EQUITY NOTE

This is not an exhaustive work, but rather a strong, supportive resource in the ongoing journey towards equity within the skin health and wellness industry.

FREE GIFT FOR YOU

"3 Reasons Why Popping That Pimple is The Last Thing You Want To Do"!

To get your FREE PRO Guide visit
www.skintheologian.com

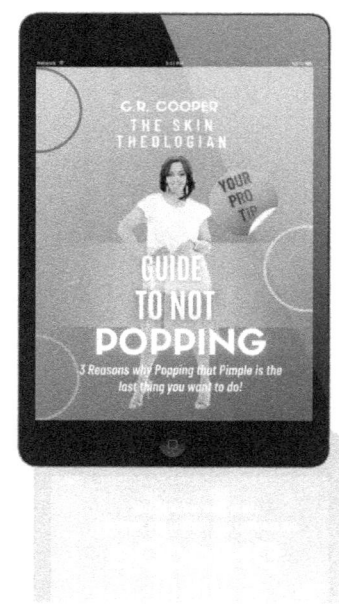

INTRODUCTION

The beauty and skincare industry is huge. It's worth billions of dollars across the globe, there's an immense choice of products out there and there are countless blogs, social media channels and videos dedicated to informing us about skincare.

It's never been easier to gather information, try out products and follow trends. But what's missing is knowing whether or not you're following the right guidance for *your* skin.

Everyone's skin is different. We react to things differently, see success in a variety of ways and have completely different skin concerns. It's the largest organ of the body and plays a critical role in the way we look and feel, as well as how our body is protected.

Education is the only way that we can understand more about our skin on a personal level. We might think we know about the basics of our skin, and how to take care of it, but think back - has anyone ever *really* told you how to care for your skin? Has anyone ever taken the time to explain the physiology of your skin, which product types you should use and a step by step of how to use them?

Or have you had to learn by yourself through trial, error and research?

As a skin professional with more than 25 years in the industry, I want to help you to learn about your skin. I want you to learn how to take care of it, give you the ability to separate fact from fiction and to ensure that you're treating your skin in the very best way that you can.

I've met many people of color who simply don't know who to trust when it comes to taking advice. For every bit of helpful advice that you receive, there's a maze of myths that you need to successfully navigate through.

I've met scores of other skincare professionals who excel at what they do, yet are nervous when it comes to treating black skin. Black skin is also woefully underrepresented in dermatology textbooks and research, which can make it difficult to get a diagnosis or recognize a condition on *your own skin.*

Studies have shown that as many as 47% of dermatologists and dermatology residents admitted that they weren't properly trained on skin conditions in black people. This can lead to inequalities in care, late diagnosis and skin conditions that aren't recognized or are treated incorrectly. Black dermatologists are underrepresented within the industry, which means that people with first-hand experience of black skin aren't the ones giving advice and guidance.

This clearly needs to be addressed so that we can receive the correct advice from professionals who are experienced in and feel confident in treating black skin effectively.

If these professionals aren't even able to recognize the way that certain skin conditions and concerns present themselves in black skin, then there's no way they can give treatment advice that's appropriate for your skin. If you're told "I don't know if that will work for you", then that's not good enough.

It's only through representation and diversity that we'll reach a fully-inclusive and understanding skincare community. It's essential that skincare professionals can treat, inform and provide guidance on all skin types, tones and concerns.

All black skin is different. It has different needs, conditions and concerns and needs different approaches as a result. Whilst there are similarities that are consistent throughout black skin, everyone's skin will have completely different, individual needs.

There are lots of us mistreating our skin, whether we're aware of it or not. Skin bleaching remains rife in the black community. It removes the precious melanin from your skin (or affects the melanin production in your skin), causing an unnatural colour, and is extremely damaging for the structure and function of your skin. But more on that later.

There is so much misleading information out there about black skin - and it comes from everywhere - that it's no surprise that people get confused about what they should be doing to take care of their skin. During my career, and even in my own experience growing up, I discovered that many black women and men are left feeling confused about their skin due to conflicting information, or information that's just completely wrong.

Let's start with something I hear all the time:

"Black don't crack!"

While it's true that black skin shows signs of aging at a slower rate than lighter skin, black skin definitely *does* crack if you don't take care of it. And unfortunately, many of us aren't taking proper care of our skin because of that information.

Here are the facts:

Black skin is susceptible to the same types of damage as other types of skin. Age spots, mottling and lentigines are all signs that your skin is aging. The timescales might be a little different when it comes to black skin compared to fairer skins, but I can assure you that over time you will develop wrinkles, sagging skin and dullness. It's a normal part of aging and happens to everyone.

You may find that dark spots and hyperpigmentation become more prevalent as you get older. The cells responsible for our melanin production are more prone to inflammation or injury. You might find that your skin has more spots than someone with lighter skin.

So in short, black *can* "crack". It might just take a bit longer than other types of skin.

It's time to dispel major myths about black skin and replace fear with confidence so that we can understand our skin and move forward in its care.

Let's level up your skincare knowledge.

WHO AM I?

C.R. Cooper - Skin Theologian

I'm a skincare professional, black woman and your Skin Theologian, here to help you navigate your skincare needs.

I have over 25 years of experience as a skin professional, working as an Education Manager and master Educator for a renowned global Skin Institute. When it comes to skin, I've seen *everything* and taught countless other skincare professionals around the world, hearing their experiences and concerns.

Day to day, I hear the same messages from both clients and other industry professionals: they're concerned about how darker skin is treated. They feel that there's inadequacies there - from the products they use to the advice they're given.

I'll be sharing feedback, comments and experiences from skincare professionals around the world throughout this book. This way, you'll be able to get behind-the-scenes, expert insights on the issues affecting your skin - as well as solutions on how to deal with them.

I love empowering people to succeed in their skincare journey or their career as a skincare professional. It all starts with knowledge, passion and interest. Black skin is beautiful, and confidence in your skin is an essential step to cracking the skincare code.

I also have a Master's of Divinity in Theology, which is where my expertise as your Skin Theologian comes in.

As we go through this book, I'll be sharing some truths with you about skin care as well as busting some myths (and there are a *lot*) along the way. I'm going to be 100% honest with you, and I won't sugarcoat the facts that you need to know, but I'll never judge.

Most of us have had to find our own way with skincare, and to work out what's best through trial and error. I'm here to help take that trial and error away with my years of experience as a skin professional.

1

SKIN THEOLOGY

In this chapter, you'll learn about:

- Skin Theology (and my take on that)
- Basic skin physiology
- Skin types, conditions and your natural skin barrier
- Black skin and the beauty industry

WHAT IS "SKIN THEOLOGY"?

In its broadest sense, theology focuses on the beliefs, rituals and commitment of different cultures throughout the world. As a skin professional with that knowledge of theology, I'm here to combine the two and bring you the structure, guidance and information that you need to take care of your skin.

Throughout the course of this book, I'll use my years of real-life experience in the skincare industry, as a black woman and as someone who speaks to skin professionals on a daily basis.

At the end of the book, you'll find my 10 Commandments for Black Skin - the rules you should take into consideration when it comes to your skin, and provide a quick reference guide if you want a reminder of what you should be doing when it comes to your skin.

There are no hidden agendas here. Just clear, honest facts to help you on your journey to understand black skin. I want to give you the necessary knowledge that you need to be able to care for black skin.

We'll start with the theory behind skincare, and the basics that you need to know to understand your skin and to help it to thrive. The theory behind the theology, if you will.

BACK TO BASICS - GET TO KNOW YOUR SKIN

The skin is the largest organ of the human body (fun fact: your skin has a total area of about 20 square feet). It protects us from germs, microbes, dirt and the elements as well as helping to regulate body temperature. It also permits us to feel sensations like touch, heat and cold.

Your skin has three layers:

- Epidermis - the outer layer of skin that provides a waterproof barrier and creates our skin tone.
- Dermis - this contains tough connective tissue, hair follicles and sweat glands. It's located just under the epidermis.
- Hypodermis - deeper subcutaneous layer that contains fat and connective tissue.

The colour of your skin is created by cells called melanocytes (located in the epidermis) which produce the pigment melanin. If you haven't heard of melanin, then you've definitely made the right decision in reading this book!

In short, melanin is a skin pigment that's responsible for making hair, skin and eyes appear darker. There are two types of melanin - eumelanin and pheomelanin. In general, the more eumelanin your skin contains, the darker your skin will be. Black skin contains more melanin than lighter skin.

The melanin in your skin is what can make it vulnerable to hyperpigmentation or dark spots. A skin breakout or damage can lead to inflammation, which in turn stimulates pigmentation.

Melanin isn't just responsible for pigment either. It also plays an important biological role by providing protection from damage from the sun. But you'd better not skip that sunscreen - if you've ever been told that you don't need SPF because of your skin color, think again!

MYTHBUSTING WITH THE SKIN THEOLOGIAN

MYTH: "I don't need to use sunscreen, my skin has natural UV protection from melanin."

TRUTH: Whilst it's true that black skin has more UV protection than other skin types, it's certainly not safe from sun damage and the risks associated with it. It's recommended that everyone - regardless of skin color - uses sunscreen with an SPF of at least 30.

You can, and will, get sunburnt in high sunshine. This can lead to skin damage and pain so cover up and wear sunscreen. Even if you don't burn - and believe me, people with darker skin *can* burn in the hot sun - you could still be causing damage to your skin.

Sunscreen is essential for all skin tones to reduce the risk of skin cancer, as well as the appearance of premature wrinkles and darkening hyperpigmentation.

Getting sunburned increases these risks. Even if you don't think you're at risk because of your melanin, you can still burn in the sun. In darker skin tones, the redness usually associated with sunburn in lighter skin can be less noticeable or even appear purplish than red. Your skin will also feel warmer, there will be pain or tenderness in the sunburned area, tightness to skin, sensitivity to touch plus tiny bumps or a rash. You'll also likely experience swelling, possibly blistering and your skin will start to peel.

If you feel discomfort, stop sun exposure immediately. This can all be mitigated by wearing around 2 teaspoons of sunscreen for face, head and arms and reapplying throughout the day.

SKIN TYPES

Your skin type is essentially the skin you were born with. If you used no products, had no routine and just let your skin do whatever it wanted...that's your skin type.

Let's do a quick round up of the four main skin types:

- **Dry Skin** - produces less sebum (the oily substance that your skin makes to help waterproof) than other skin types, which can leave your skin feeling tight and looking . dull. As your skin isn't very moisturized naturally, you'll need to add moisture back in to protect your natural skin barrier.
- **Oily Skin** - this skin type over-produces sebum leaving skin looking shiny and even appearing

thickened. May have large pores, blackheads and spots as a result of sebum getting trapped in pores.
- **Normal Skin** - relatively balanced, normal skin that contains the right mix of sebum and moisturizing factors. Pore size and skin texture isn't an issue.
- **Combination Skin** - a mixture of skin types that usually manifests as a greasier T-Zone (forehead and nose) or areas like your cheeks.

MYTHBUSTING WITH THE SKIN THEOLOGIAN

MYTH: "Black skin is oily."

TRUTH: Black skin comes in all different types. Whilst some black skin will be oily, other black skin may be prone to dryness (or a combination of the two). You need to use the right products and routines for your skin type.

The skin on your face can have different needs to the skin on your body - you can have dry skin on one and oily on the other, so be prepared to use products for different skin types on your face and body.

Skin can also be sensitive in addition to any of these skin types, which can be genetic or caused by external factors such as products. Dry skin tends to be more prone to becoming sensitive, as your skin's natural barrier is usually damaged.

SKIN CONDITIONS

A skin condition is something going on with your skin that usually relates to lifestyle factors or genetics. Skin conditions may be temporary or longer term. We'll go into more detail later on in the book about building a skin routine that's right for your individual skin type and conditions, including how to treat some conditions (and when it's time to speak to a professional).

Common skin condition that can affect any type of skin include:

Acne

A long-term skin condition that occurs when dead skin cells and oil from the skin cloghair follicles. This is characterized by blackheads or whiteheads, pimples and oily skin. Acne can cause scarring on all skin types, but on black skin this can cause hyperpigmentation and dark spots which can be more visible than the acne itself.

You also need to be careful about which products you use on your skin - or which medication you take - when dealing with acne as some very common products can also exacerbate hyperpigmentation (more on that later).

Black skin tends to suffer from inflammatory acne, which luckily, is the easiest type of acne to treat. The treatment involved in managing acne in black skin is no different to the treatment used in other skin types/races but black people tend to have fewer nodules and cysts.

Aging

Everyone's skin ages. That's a fact. The passing of time happens to everyone and brings a loss of collagen and elasticity (leading to sagging skin), fine lines and wrinkles, age spots and loss of facial volume. Your skin may get drier as you age.

It's all completely normal. Whilst it's true that black skin can show signs of aging less quickly than other skin types, your skin will still get older, just as you will.

Dehydration

Dehydrated skin commonly gets confused with dry skin. Any skin type - even oily - can be dehydrated, which is where your skin is temporarily low on water. It's completely fixable. Dry skin is a permanent skin type, where your skin is low on oil, not water.

Dehydration is often caused by low humidity, hot showers, heating and not getting enough water.

Dermatosis Papulosa Nigra

This condition is way more common in black skins. It presents as small, benign skin lesions and bumps together on the skin. They're thought to be genetic and cause no harm, but many people dislike their appearance and may look to have them removed. Scarring, hyperpigmentation and keloids can all be a potential side-effect of removal, so it's essential that you speak to someone who is experienced in black skin if you're investigating removal.

Around one third of the black population experiences Dermatosis Papulosa Nigra as they age, making it a common skin condition within the black community.

Eczema

Eczema can be inherited or through reacting to something in your environment. It causes an itchy red rash that comes on gradually and can last a long time. It's triggered by things like stress, temperature changes, allergies or dry skin.

It can occur anywhere on the body but is most common in areas such as the inside of the elbows, back of the knees, face, behind the ears, buttocks, hands and feet.

It's believed to occur twice as frequently in children with darker skin. Often, eczema is misdiagnosed when it comes to black skin. This means that treatment is slow or non-existent which then can cause issues with pigmentation.

Ichthyosis

This genetic skin condition is characterized by dry, thickened and scaly skin. It ranges in severity, symptoms and the underlying genetic cause. It can be itchy, dry and painful.

Keratosis Pilaris

This commonly goes hand in hand with eczema and ichthyosis. It gives the appearance of goosebumps (or 'chicken skin'), most commonly around thighs and the tops of your arms. It isn't painful or contagious, but can be annoying. It's your hair follicles producing too much keratin.

Melasma

This condition is often linked with pregnancy, but it can also appear in men and women who aren't pregnant (usually over the age of 40). It usually consists of large patches of discoloration on the face and cheeks, often on the high points of the face like the cheeks, bridge of the nose, forehead and upper lip. It can be caused by hormone treatments, medication, sun exposure and pregnancy and is prevalent in women of color.

Pigmentation

We've already talked about this a little but pigmentation can be a problem for darker skins. Whether it's sun damage, scarring, acne or a hormonal condition, darker skin can show pigmentation more visibly than other skin types. Be careful with treatment as some products and treatments can cause further pigmentation to your skin - more on that to come.

Pityriasis Alba

Pityriasis Alba mostly affects black children on their face and arms but it has been known to appear on other areas of the body. In this instance, scaly patches of skin that are round and light in colour form. Unlike other conditions like vitiligo, the colour change is temporary and disappears after treatment has been applied.

Psoriasis

Psoriasis is an autoimmune condition that causes inflammation as well as dry, red, itchy and scaly skin. It usually appears in patches, often concentrated around the elbows, knees, lower back and scalp. It usually needs medical attention and prescription treatment to be resolved, so speak to your doctor or dermatologist.

Rosacea

Rosacea is another auto-inflammatory skin condition. It has a range of different "levels" and over time is becoming more common in darker skin tones. It's easily missed on black skin by both medical professionals and people with the condition, as it was thought that darker skins don't experience rosacea.

This isn't the case, and the great news is that there's increasing awareness of how the condition presents itself in darker skin. If your face constantly feels warm or flushed, burns or strings, discolours, has dry patches that appear swollen or have acne-type spots that don't clear up with treatment then it's worth investigating whether or not you have rosacea. You may also experience swollen, thickened skin or hardened bumps around the mouth or eyes, as well as sensitivity to skin products.

Vitiligo

Signs of vitiligo usually present themselves before adulthood. People with vitiligo have the same number of melanocytes (the cells that produce melanin and contribute to your skin tone) but they aren't active. This leads to patches of paler skin.

The condition is more noticeable in skin of colour and is considered to be an autoimmune condition. This condition needs treatment from a skin specialist.

SKIN THEOLOGIAN'S TIP

When it comes to skincare, treat your skin condition before your skin type. Skin conditions can mask your skin type, and make it harder to treat. This may mean prioritizing some skin products over others.

OTHER SKIN CONCERNS FOR BLACK SKIN

As well as skin conditions, there are some other skin concerns that can affect black skin more prominently than other skin types. These can include:

Ashy skin

Dry skin occurs in every type of skin, but it's way more noticeable with black skin. It can leave skin looking a little grey, dry and flaky. This can make it difficult to apply makeup and products on your skin.

Hyperpigmentation

Also known as Post-Inflammatory Hyperpigmentation (PIH). This usually happens if the skin has experienced some form of trauma such as insect bites, acne, burns or surgical cuts. As the skin heals, the wounded area appears darker in colour. These dark spots and scars do eventually heal but it can affect confidence and lead to people taking extreme measures to "fix" the problem. These "fixes" can often make it worse.

Lichenification

This is a harmless condition but is often the result of other skin conditions such as eczema or dermatitis. Lichenification can be caused by stress and consists of excessive itching or rubbing, resulting in an irritable rash. It is treatable and the skin can return to normal once the inflammation is kept under control but it can be difficult to identify in black skin and is often confused with fungal infections.

Keloid scars

Keloid scars are raised scarring on the skin that may have discoloration, redness or irritation. It's your body's overreaction to wound healing through the production of too many fibroblasts in your skin. This is why people with black skin need to be really careful with acne, piercings or anything else that might leave a scar or dark spots behind it. Your skin cells can go crazy, leaving scarring in its wake.

Razor burn

We'll run through this in more detail later, but because of the texture and coil of black hair, razor burn, ingrown hairs and bumps can be more prevalent in black skin. Because of the curl pattern of the hair, hair can curl back on itself underneath the skin and cause an ingrown hair. This can lead to discomfort, infection and later, discoloration. Most common in men who need to shave

As you can see, black skin comes with its own range of issues that your routine and lifestyle needs to support. Good skin doesn't just happen by accident, it's about being consistent and purposeful with your beauty routines.

YOUR SKIN BARRIER

Your skin barrier is the outside layer of your skin that protects your body from the environment, as well as balancing out the water in your body. Your skin barrier is invisible, and as long as you're treating it well, you shouldn't even really be able to tell that it's there. It'll just be protecting with no cause for concern.

If you've been neglecting your skin (not drinking enough water, using overly harsh products etc.) then your skin barrier can become damaged and you'll experience dry skin, itching and inflammation. You might struggle with products 'disappearing' from your skin, and tight skin that 'drinks' up your moisturizer in no time at all, leaving skin quickly feeling dry again.

The good news is that it can be repaired if it is damaged, but it's way easier just to take care of it in the first place than trying to restore the delicate balance from scratch.

In black skin, your skin barrier can be more prone to water loss (due to having less ceramides in the skin) which can make your skin feel rough or dry.

QUICK TRUTHS: THE STRUCTURE OF BLACK SKIN AND CONDITIONS

We'll go into more detail about the ins and outs of darker skin later in the book, but here are some facts-on-the-go to help you to understand your skin better:

- The epidermis isn't thicker in black skin, but is instead more compact. This is great news for the tone and elasticity of your skin.
- The skin barrier of darker skin can be more prone to losing moisture thanks to a process called trans-epidermal water loss (TEWL) which means skin can feel rough and dry
- Black skin is more prone to hyperpigmentation
- Keloid scarring - thick, raised and dark scars at the site of trauma, body modification or burns - is more prevalent in black skin
- Flesh moles can be more common in black skin
- Dryness on black skin manifests as ashiness

You need to be aware of the issues that can face black skin tones so that you can deal with them, or prevent them, effectively.

MYTHBUSTING WITH THE SKIN THEOLOGIAN

MYTH: "Black skin is thicker than other skin types."

TRUTH: This is a worrying misconception that stems from cruel experimentation hundreds of years ago. Unfortunately, its legacy still lives on in up to a third of medical professionals, leading to poor treatment options for a range of skin and medical conditions.

Black skin isn't thicker than other skin types. It has some natural protection from UV rays and a more compact epidermis, which can benefit the tone and elasticity of the skin.

THE BEAUTY INDUSTRY AND BLACK SKIN

Despite the fact that black women spend almost 10 times as much money on beauty products than their white counterparts, the beauty of black skin has been traditionally excluded from mainstream media, beauty launches and skincare products. Where it has been included, it has sometimes felt inauthentic.

Unfortunately this creates a vicious cycle where skin of color isn't considered during the development, creation or marketing stages of new products. Products across the entire beauty industry are being created with Eurocentric notions of beauty attached to them, without considering the needs of black skin.

It spans the entire industry, from product research and development right through to products being on the shelves. Starting with products that aren't developed with black skin in mind, or tested on different skin tones right from the beginning, right through to photoshoots that don't feature anyone with black skin, filled with make up artists and hair stylists that don't have the right products. No-one wants to look gray on a shoot.

Make up ranges regularly don't feature a full spectrum of tones, or an acknowledgement of what products might look like on black skin. The fact is: it's gonna look different. Brands would do much better sales-wise if they showed that.

Often, in "mainstream" beauty retailers, there's a shelf dedicated to specific beauty products aimed at black consumers. In books, articles and magazines black skin sometimes gets a paragraph (if it even gets mentioned at all). There are a lot of us, and we have skincare needs! It's not enough that we have to rely on passing around information like it's a secret.

A side effect of this lack of representation is that we have to rely on trial-and-error or word-of-mouth recommendations to find products that are suitable for our skin. It's more difficult than just being able to head into any drug store anywhere and pick up a product that we know will be correct for skin of color.

This is definitely improving. Each year there are more and more skin care products and ranges being created with the needs of people of color in mind, and there is more representation of beautiful black skin in the mainstream media than ever before.

There are still issues with ingredients, color ranges for makeup and representation of diversity in the media. Only we can change that, by becoming a voice to be heard and represented within the industry.

KEY TAKEAWAYS

- Darker skin contains more melanin than lighter skin tones.
- There are some skin conditions that can be more prevalent in black skin than in other types of skin.
- Black skin needs SPF. Period.
- Black skin isn't thicker than other skin types.
- Not all products will be right for your skin, or designed with black skin in mind.

2

THE SKIN PRO'S PERSPECTIVE

In this chapter, you'll learn about:

- What skincare professionals really think about black skin
- Whether you actually do need a skincare professional
- How to find a skincare professional that's right for you
- Some tips for what to look out for when you're working with a skincare professional

LEAVE IT TO THE PROFESSIONALS...RIGHT?

One of the best ways to learn - about anything, not just skin - is from the professionals. The beauty industry is filled with experts who really *know* about skin.

Something that I've noticed from my own experience in the industry, and the experiences of clients and contacts, is that sometimes the professionals aren't as well-versed in working with black skin. They may even be a little nervous about how to handle it, believing that anything they do with black skin will lead to darker pigmentation or damage.

They may not have been taught to recognize certain skin conditions and how they present differently in black skin. They may have never seen an image of a skin concern on black skin in a textbook, let alone in person. This becomes another cycle as because they're not experienced in black skin, they shy away from treating it.

It's a fact that only 3% of dermatologists in the US are black, which leads to disparities in diagnosis and treatment of skin conditions and concerns. These may present differently in black skin, in a way that's rarely seen in medical textbooks.

Location and clientele all play their part in the cycle too. If you never have clients with darker skin tones, you don't get the opportunity to learn and enhance your practical knowledge, which in turn affects confidence about treating darker skin.

Against a backdrop of limited training, this can all add up.

This lack of experience in black skin from skin care professionals can lead to:

- Bad advice that can be damaging for the skin
- Ineffective routines, treatments and product recommendations
- A lack of trust in beauty and skincare professionals

LET'S GET DIRECT: SKIN CARE PROFESSIONALS AND BLACK SKIN

I decided to go straight to the source (would I even be the Skincare Theologian if I wasn't all about discovery?) and speak to senior skin professionals from around the world to find out their thoughts on black skin care.

These professionals come from a range of different backgrounds, roles in the industry and completely different perspectives. They're based all around the world, in metropolitan and rural areas. Some head up education departments of skin care companies some own and run salons, some head up beauty brands, others are trained skin professionals with years of experience.

Their opinions are essential when it comes to skincare for black and darker skin tones. They matter, and their experiences are likely to be representative of the wider industry as a whole. I am deeply grateful for their participation in this research, without which we would not have these important industry insights.

So, what did I ask these skincare professionals? I kept it simple and top-level, asking them the most pertinent questions to gauge where they're at when it comes to black skin. I asked them about their experiences and knowledge of working with black skin, including:

1. **In your experience, what's the top concern with black skin?**
2. **What's the number one myth with black skin?**
3. **What do you think black clients lack when it comes to adequate skincare?**
4. **BONUS QUESTION: On a scale of 1-10 (10 being highly confident), how confident are you in treating clients with black and darker skin?**

LET'S TALK ABOUT THE RESULTS

We asked the professionals the questions above and collated their responses. Many of the answers and trends we observed echoed my own findings as a black skin care professional. I wouldn't necessarily say there were any big surprises, but more a confirmation of some of the trends and themes that I've observed in the industry during my decades of experience.

So, let's take a deep dive into the survey responses, what they show us and what insights we can take to further improve the advice, guidance and confidence within the industry when it comes to working with black skin.

The responses have been sectioned by question. We've provided an analysis of the most common responses and will go into more detail about some of the responses received in the survey.

1. In your experience, what's the top concern with black skin?

Absolutely no surprises here! The biggest concern reported by skincare professionals when it comes to black skin is **hyperpigmentation**. Whether that's Post Inflammatory Pigmentation (PIH), discoloration, melasma or uneven pigmentation.

Over 80% of responses to the survey mentioned hyperpigmentation in black skin.

It was also mentioned that there's often a focus on treating the hyperpigmentation itself rather than preventing the causes of the hyperpigmentation in the first place. Especially when it comes to dark marks left by acne, eczema, sun exposure or inflammation.

Concerns around identifying skin conditions and or redness on black skins were also raised, as were the perceptions that black skin can be dehydrated, oily or both. Others in the survey mentioned folliculitis from shaving in black men and pigmentation issues from ingrown hairs.

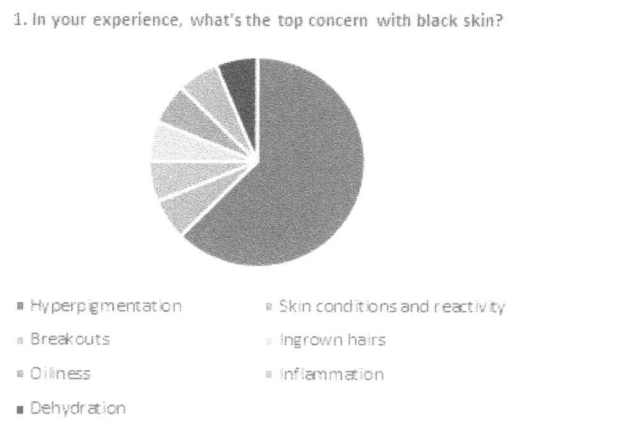

1. In your experience, what's the top concern with black skin?

- Hyperpigmentation
- Breakouts
- Oiliness
- Dehydration
- Skin conditions and reactivity
- Ingrown hairs
- Inflammation

2. What's the number one myth with black skin?

Again, this probably won't come as any surprise! The number one misconception that skin professionals reported when it comes to black skin is the perception that black skin doesn't get damaged by the sun, doesn't need SPF and that black skin is somehow immune to skin cancer.

66% of skin care professionals that we surveyed mentioned 'not needing sunscreen' as the number one myth they heard regularly about black skin.

You will probably have heard these sentiments before in your own life. It's a long-held belief by many people, black and otherwise.

Yes, your skin has more melanin which gives more natural protection for your skin than other skin tones.

No, this doesn't mean you have natural all-round sun protection, whatever the weather. The sun's UV rays can still damage your skin if you're black, and skin cancer doesn't discriminate based on skin colour.

I'm going to say it again (louder for the people in the back!) - **black skin needs sun protection. Your skin can be damaged by the sun, and black skin can be affected by skin cancer.**

MYTHBUSTING WITH THE SKIN THEOLOGIAN

MYTH: "Sunscreen makes black skin look ashy."

TRUTH: *Some* sunscreen makes black skin look ashy or gray as it has a white cast to it. Zinc sunscreens can be challenging for this, which is unfortunate as it's one of the most effective ingredients for sun protection. A mineral sunscreen (like zinc) provides better sun protection and is less likely to cause allergies.

I'm not going to recommend specific brands or products here as I want this book to give you unbiased, useful knowledge that you can use to help you make your own decisions and choices about skincare.

But, there are good-quality sunscreens out there that have been specifically formulated with black skin in mind and won't leave a white cast on your skin. Look them up, your skin will thank you for it.

Some of the other common myths that were highlighted in the survey responses included:

- Black skin is somehow stronger than other skin types and doesn't experience sensitivity (which can then lead to damage and hyperpigmentation)
- That you can't see redness or sensitivity on black skin
- That black skin needs handled completely differently to all other types of skin
- Black skin that's oily doesn't need a moisturizer
- All black skin is oily

Do any of these myths sound familiar to you? Yep, me too.

Needless to say, all of them are myths. Black skin isn't stronger and can experience redness and sensitivity. Whilst black skin needs to be treated differently in some ways, overall, it's just skin and has the same physiological make up, structure and needs as other types of skin.

Black skin isn't always oily either - it can be dehydrated and oily at the same time, just like other types of skin - and even if it is oily, you need moisturizer to hydrate and protect it.

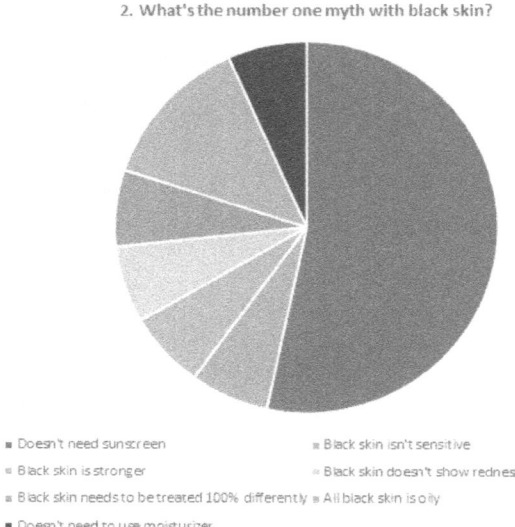

2. What's the number one myth with black skin?

- Doesn't need sunscreen
- Black skin isn't sensitive
- Black skin is stronger
- Black skin doesn't show redness
- Black skin needs to be treated 100% differently
- All black skin is oily
- Doesn't need to use moisturizer

3. What do you think black clients lack when it comes to adequate skincare?

First of all, notice the question I asked was around *adequate* skincare. Not "amazing" or "the best" or "top-tier" skincare. Adequate. As in the *minimum* that you should expect when it comes to skincare.

The main response from the skin professionals was that black clients lacked the right education around skincare and the right products. This is definitely something that many of us with black skin have experienced, left to rely on word-of-mouth recommendations or trial and error to work out what's best.

Again, this answer wasn't wholly surprising to me as a black skin care professional. The whole reason for writing this book was a lack of specific, focused skincare advice for black skin from the industry.

There's always an element of trying out a product to decide whether or not you'll actually like it but it shouldn't always need to be trial and error to see if you need it in the first place.

So, whether it's use of laser treatments on black skin (more on that later), working out the right peels, dealing with hyperpigmentation or other concerns like eczema or acne. We aren't always aware of what's best for our skin, and what's suitable. If we aren't getting that information from the professionals either...then where are we meant to get it from?

A lack of professional estheticians who are experienced in black skin (yep), as well as keloid scarring and dehydration were other issues mentioned in relation to the pieces that are missing in the skincare puzzle for black clients.

3. What do you think black clients lack when it comes to adequate skincare?

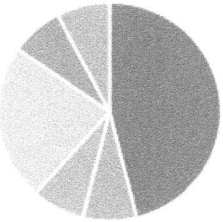

- Education on the right skincare
- How to avoid inflammation
- Sunscreen that doesn't turn ashy
- Product recommendation
- How to avoid dryness
- Keloid scarring

4. BONUS QUESTION: On a scale of 1-10 (10 being highly confident), how confident are you in treating clients with black and darker skin?

For me, this was a *really* important question to ask. It required honesty and candour from the skincare professionals who completed the survey and I think that's what we got. I really appreciate that, as we need more open conversations with professionals and individuals to start moving forward and enjoying our best skin.

Let's take a deeper dive into how this question was answered and what issues this raises for us to delve into a little further. Here we go...

On average, the **skincare professionals we asked rated themselves as a 7.5 out of 10** when it came to knowledge and confidence in treating black skin. This was a relief to hear.

However, based on experience, it has come to mind that the skin professionals we spoke to are just that - experienced professionals, mostly used to treating all manner of skin types - so they may actually be more knowledgeable than the average skincare practitioner. This is less of a relief if you think about it in those terms. We asked experts, and they said that (on average) they were 7.5 out of 10 confident in treating black skin - absolutely no shade here, but where does that leave the rest of the industry who *aren't* experts?

Location and client base played a big part in the answers to this question. It isn't a shock that the skincare professionals who regularly treat black skin felt more confident about it. In parts of the world where there's less diversity, confidence was lower. This is part of that cycle again where without black clients, you don't feel comfortable in treating black skin, which means you don't get black clients. And so it continues on and on.

Over 25% of the skincare professionals we asked rated themselves as 10 out of 10 when it came to confidence. They have a variety of clients with different skin types and are comfortable treating all of them, or they have a client base that predominantly has black skin so are totally comfortable in handling darker skin tones..

Here's a snippet of some of the comments that the survey unearthed from those who felt totally confident in their treatment of black skin:

"I have lots of black clients."

"I'm very confident working with black or darker complexions. There are still a lot of misconceptions about black skin - around SPF and tanning in particular."

"I feel very confident that I can provide high-quality treatment to all types of skin."

A further **41% rated themselves a 7, 8 or a 9** when it came to confidence on treating black skin. We'd say this rating is still good, but shows that there needs to be a little more work in just nudging that confidence a little higher.

It's definitely all positive and shows that overall, **66% of the skin care professionals that we asked felt confident about treating black skin.** Though some did acknowledge that this still meant that they were less confident about black skin than other skin types (for example, rating themselves as a 10 out 10 for their confidence and knowledge of Caucasian skin vs a lower rating of their confidence in treating black skin).

Here's a snippet of some of the comments that the survey unearthed from those who felt relatively confident in their treatment of black skin:

> *"That's the majority of my clients. I don't always know everything so I'm always learning and communicating with colleagues, reps and manufacturers to find out more."*

> *"I have lots of experience with black and Asian skins. Sometimes these clients have gone to extreme lengths for their complexion."*

> *"There's still so much I need to learn."*

> *"My knowledge of black skin is just slightly lower than my knowledge of lighter skin."*

Unfortunately, around **33% of the skin care professionals rated their confidence in treating black skin as 6 out of 10 or lower**.

This is something of a concern, although if I'm being really honest, probably not that much of a surprise again. We've experienced it, lived it and heard about it all too often. It's disappointing to see.

Here's a snippet of some of the comments that the survey unearthed from those who didn't feel confident in their knowledge and confidence in treating black skin:

> *"I would say I feel confident about the physiology of the skin. But as someone with light skin I'm not always sure I have enough knowledge to meet cultural or specific understanding of the needs of clients with darker skin."*

> *"I have experience in working with Asian clients, but not clients with black skin - I just haven't had the clients to learn on."*
> *"In the US overall, I would say that it's about 5 out of*

10 when it comes to getting advice for black skin. It does depend on training though."

"During my training I had no clients with black skin. There are so many misconceptions about black skin and a lack of both knowledge and accessible information in Australia."

This means that as a black woman or man, when you step into the salon, store or somewhere else where you're looking for that much-needed expertise, you **have a 1 in 3 chance of someone giving you skincare advice - or even performing a skin treatment on you - when they are not confident about treating black skin.**

Not only can this leave you dissatisfied and perpetuate the ongoing cycle of a lack of proper skincare advice, it could cause damage to your skin.

Black skin is not something that professionals should be intimidated by. This needs to change.

DO YOU EVEN NEED TO VISIT A SKINCARE PROFESSIONAL?

In my (professional) opinion, yes. Working with the right skin care professional can make a world of difference to your skin -

especially if you have particular concerns that need to be addressed with specialist treatment.

Many skin conditions or issues won't go away on their own. Treating them at home when you don't necessarily have the right expertise, tools or products can be a recipe for disaster. You can make them worse, or cause further damage to your skin. Nobody wants that.

What I'm definitely *not* saying is that you can never, ever do anything with your own skin and must leave it in the hands of a professional at all times. Come on, it's skin - it's *your* skin - and you know it best.

What I am saying is that for the most part, skincare professionals go through years of training to become experts in skin. They've usually seen it all, and by choosing the right match for your skin, they can help you to achieve your skincare goals.

Some people are lucky and just have skin that behaves itself throughout their life. Not all of us are so lucky. Whether we do or don't have naturally "good" skin, a professional can help you to find out more about your skin and what you can do to make every day your best skin day.

The other great thing about visiting a skincare professional is that it can be considered a form of self-care. It's time for yourself that focuses on you and making you look and feel your best. It's an investment in both your inner and outer beauty, that you absolutely deserve.

Skincare treatments aren't for everyone. Some people just don't enjoy them or don't get the benefits they're looking for from their treatments. This could be because it's just not something that's for you, or it could be that you're not working with the right skincare professional. If this is you, I'd still recommend that you maintain a good skincare regime at home.

If you suspect it's the latter, the next section might just be what you're looking for.

FINDING A SKIN PROFESSIONAL WHO KNOWS ABOUT BLACK SKIN

Getting it right when it comes to your skin is *so* important. It's worth putting in the work to find the right skin care professional for you (and your skin). It might take a little longer to do the groundwork, but the results will be worth it.

Instead of ineffective advice or a tentative approach that leaves you frustrated or disappointed, you'll get advice and guidance that really does take *your skin* into account. A good skincare professional will take the time to get to know you, your circumstances, any skincare concerns and your skincare goals.

Here are the steps that you should take when looking for your perfect skincare match:

1. Work out what you need

An esthetician is different to a dermatologist. Dermatologists are medically trained and can diagnose, prescribe and give medical advice - as a rule of thumb, if it's a skin abnormality, disorder or severe skin reaction then it's a dermatologist that you're probably looking for. The same if you're looking for more invasive or medical treatments like fillers, botox or other 'tweakments'

Estheticians focus more on skincare routines, routine procedures (such as facials or peels) and can give advice on achieving skincare goals. You can get medical estheticians who focus more on treatments like light therapy, lasers, chemical peels and helping with recovery from skincare issues like burns. Then there are more generalised estheticians, who can still deliver a skincare routine - they tend to work at spas and salons.

2. Do your research

I can't emphasize this *enough*. Seek out those recommendations, read those reviews and search whatever your social media of choice is to find the right skin care professional for you.

Treat it like dating, treat it like a job interview, treat it like finding the best restaurant for your birthday. This is important, and spending more time on research now will stop you wasting your time in the future.

3. Have a consultation

A skin professional worth their weight in active ingredients will be happy to have a consultation with you to understand your needs and the needs of your skin. There might be a cost involved for the consultation but it really could be money well-spent.

Virtual consultations have become much more popular over recent years, and these can be much more convenient and cost-effective.

During the consultation process, ask questions. What's their experience, who are their clients, do they understand what black skin needs? Did they ask about your current regimen? Have they asked about your lifestyle? What products do they use? Check out their qualifications and keep an eye on cleanliness. If they're not the right fit, then ok. You can move on, and head back to the research phase.

4. Trust your instincts

After you leave your consultation, pause and just replay the consultation. Trust your instincts about how you feel. Were they professional? Did they say anything that set off your warning lights? Did they recommend a 25-step regiment when you told them you only have 10 minutes max for skincare in the morning? Did you actually like them, or at least gel with them?

We aren't saying you have to be besties, but having a skincare professional that you can trust is important.

5. Don't be afraid to speak up

A good skincare professional should listen to you. You're paying for their expertise, but as the client they need to listen to you too. Don't be made to feel that you don't know your own skin, and if you need to move on, then you can.

It's been proven that there are misconceptions around black skin and pain tolerance. Pain should never be part of the process (without warning or support).

SKIN THEOLOGIAN'S TIP

When it comes to finding skincare professionals who are used to treating black skin, there are all the usual ways of finding recommendations.

However, more and more specific groups are being formed that solely focus on recommending skincare professionals and dermatologists who know exactly what they're doing for darker skin.

Here's a selection from around the world to help you in your research:

Spasho - aimed at clients in the US, this site is a resource to connect black estheticians with clients who are looking for their expertise.

Black Skincare Directory - based in the UK, this directory acts as a starting point for skincare research and signposting towards the professionals you need in your life.

Skin of Color Society - this site provides a doctor database to connect you with dermatologists and skin specialists in the US.

Black Aesthetics Advisory Board - skincare specialists who are working together to investigate the experiences of black practitioners within aesthetics, as well as consumers.

This certainly isn't an exhaustive list (and I wish it was longer) but there are new sites cropping up and a raft of articles, recommendations and Instagram lists to help you to find the right fit for your skin.

THINGS TO BE AWARE OF WITH PROFESSIONAL SKIN CARE TREATMENTS

So you've found the ideal skincare pro. You've done your research, you're happy that they're going to be a match for your skin. They know how to treat black skin. You know what you want to discuss and you have an idea what you might need.

Your appointment is booked and you've confirmed. All super-positive and a key part of the process.

Without sounding too dramatic, it's still really important to be vigilant. I'm definitely not being down on estheticians or skincare professionals (I mean...I am one!). It's never been - and never will be - in my interests to bash anyone, least of all skincare professionals, but I've seen the damage that can be done by someone who's inexperienced with black skin. Even if they have the best of intentions.

It's easier to prevent the damage in the first place than to solve the side effects later, as is the case with most skincare to be honest! Here are some things to keep in mind when you visit a skincare professional, especially if you're having a treatment such as a facial:

Your skin should be treated with care

I get it, a harsh skin routine that gives visible results can be super-satisfying (there's a reason people watch those pimple-popping videos that are all over the internet). But because of the propensity of black skin towards hyperpigmentation, scarring and inflammation, you don't want this from a skincare professional. You just don't. With a new facialist, skincare professional or esthetician you want them to do it nice, easy and gentle until they discover what your skin can tolerate without these side-effects.

Be aware of the effects of lasers on black skin

Whether it's for hair removal, rejuvenation or pigment removal, lasers aren't always good news for black skin. Sometimes they can be ineffective (especially when it comes to hair removal) and at worst can cause damage or scarring to your skin. Different locations have different rules on who can use lasers on client skin so be aware of the rules in your region on this.

Take care with retinoids

If you're a skincare enthusiast already and are trying out a prescription-only retinoid (such as tretinoin), firstly make sure your skincare professional knows about it and is aware that you're taking this treatment. Secondly, it's usually best to skip it for a week before you have any sort of facial treatment. If you forget to stop, mention it to your skincare professional as it can make your skin more delicate, and it might be best to rebook.

Keep an eye on steaming and extractions

Both of these are mainstays of a traditional facial process but these have often not been designed with black skin in mind. Your skin can react differently, so it's best to proceed with caution and take the guidance of an experienced professional on this. DIY or at-home versions of these should be avoided (to avoid damage) in my opinion - if you make a mistake and end up damaging your skin then a professional will likely be needed to help your skin recover.

Will you need recovery time?

Again, not to be dramatic but sometimes a skin treatment can temporarily affect your skin negatively. We're thinking treatments like chemical peels that leave your skin shedding temporarily. Your skincare professional should really let you know ahead of time if this is going to be the case so that you can prepare (even if that's just by clearing your diary or limiting face to face appointments). Sometimes it's best not to have a facial right before a special occasion, just in case it makes you break out.

The finishing touches

A sign that a skincare professional isn't that well-versed in handling black skin can sometimes all be in the finishing touches.

If they apply SPF or mineral powder at the end of the treatment that leaves you looking grey or powdery...it's a no. And you can say no to this final step if you feel your skin is going to be better off without it but it's my absolute professional opinion that every professional face treatment/facial should be completed with an SPF application.

So at the very least, the skin professional should have options for you. If not, it's ok to say no then and there.

This isn't an exhaustive list but should help you on your way to finding a skin professional that understands you and your skin.

KEY TAKEAWAYS

- Some skincare professionals don't fully understand how to work with black skin. This needs to change.
- You should exercise (sensible) caution when selecting a skincare professional to work with. Not all skincare professionals are equal, especially when it comes to black skin.
- Ultimately, when it comes to your skin, you have the final say.

3

MORE THAN SKIN DEEP

*I*n this chapter, you'll learn about:

- The history of skin care
- The history of the black beauty industry
- Skin in the here and now

Let's talk more about the skin, how it's evolved over time, the history of skincare and the developments that we've made throughout the process. Along with the places where we still need work.

THE EVOLUTION OF SKIN

First of all we're going to start by combining history with a little science. As a Skin Theologian, history, storytelling and understanding beliefs, theories and purpose are part of who I am and I want to share that knowledge with you. I think context is important, even if it's a brief overview, to get a feel for where things have been, where they are and where they're going.

Anyway, back to the history of skin.

For hundreds of thousands of years, humans - or a version of today's humans, earlier versions existed millions of years before that - have existed on the planet. It's widely believed that the human population originated in Africa.

Although scientists disagree about some of the *exact* theories of whereabouts in Africa the first humans originated, there is lots of evidence to support the theory that everyone has their roots in Africa, no matter where they are in the world.

It's also thought that the first humans had dark skin, as we evolved to lose our fur (imagine that) and turned on our melanin-producing cells as a way to protect our skin from the sun (again, most animals have fur to do that) and to ensure that we could absorb and store folate, to continue to reproduce.

Also, we developed more sweat glands - which we obviously still have today - during this time to help us deal with the heat and forage for longer periods.

For most of history, humans have had dark skin. It's only when humans started to migrate to other parts of the world, such as Europe, around 200,000 years ago that they developed lighter skin. It's thought that this was to absorb more vitamin D and shed that natural UV protection to make it easier to get their vitamins from the sun's rays (but remember, *today* you still need to use SPF - no using examples from hundreds of thousands of years ago to try and get out of it).

SKIN THEOLOGIAN'S TIP

Ok, this one isn't really a tip - more of a tip-off - but if you *really* want to learn more about the origins of different types of skin in a scientific way, here are some resources to take a look at:

New gene variants reveal the evolution of skin color - Science Magazine

The Biology of Skin Color - Discover

Ancient Briton had Dark Skin and Light Eyes - Smithsonian

I'm the Skin Theologian, not the Skin Scientist (though skincare and science is often linked very closely) - sometimes this type of information is best left in the hands of those with the right scientific background.

There's a whole lot of scientific papers and research out there that delve into the history and evolution of skin in as much detail as you want to go. For the purposes of this book, we'll keep the time travel relatively top-level.

As you can see, when it comes to skin, it's actually way more than just skin deep. This stuff has been developing over hundreds of thousands - if not millions - of years and is the result of migration, chance and evolution. It really is amazing when you think about it.

Today, it's harder to pinpoint the exact percentage of the world that has black or darker skin tones. It gets complicated as people identify themselves differently throughout the world, heritages combine and how do you do an accurate study of billions of people that are scattered across the planet anyway? Maybe in the future this will be data that becomes more available.

What I do know, *without* needing a worldwide census, is that it's more than enough of the world's population who have darker skin for the beauty and skincare industry to have stepped up long before now to develop products, ingredients and treatments - as well as skincare professionals who are adept at treating black skin - for those of us with darker skin tones.

So with that, let's delve into the archives a little bit and talk more about the history of skin, skincare and the industry around it.

SKINCARE THROUGH THE AGES

Ok, time for another (brief) history lesson about our skin. Don't worry, we're not going to talk in Latin like so many theology texts, scientific papers and skincare ingredients lists do.

The anatomy of, understanding of and modification of skin has been going on for thousands and thousands of years. Medical documents that talk about skin conditions and concerns go back as far as 1500 BC (yes, *BC*, not the 1500's as in 500 years ago which itself seems like a long time ago!). It's called the Ebers Papyrus if you've got the urge to read some medical papers from Ancient Egypt in your spare time.

With that, let's start with a trip - back to the history of the African continent again - to ancient Egypt (are you ready for your Cleopatra moment?) and how they kickstarted the beauty industry around 6,000 years ago.

CLEANSE LIKE AN EGYPTIAN

Archaeological evidence has uncovered cosmetics from thousands of years ago in Ancient Egypt. But the cosmetics weren't just for aesthetic reasons, men and women used them to protect themselves from the elements (like the sun, insects and sandstorms) and to honor their gods and goddesses.

For skincare, the Ancient Egyptians used lots of ingredients that are *still used* in skincare today. They're the original skinfluencers (and were rocking the eyeliner flick way before anyone else). Some of these ingredients include castor, sesame and moringa oil to fight wrinkles as well as soap made from clay and olive oil to cleanse. Egyptian women also incorporated honey and milk masks into their skincare routine to moisturize, as well as the famous milk baths and dead sea salts to exfoliate, rejuvenate and heal their skin.

Is it just me that feels like this routine wouldn't actually be that out of place even now, 6,000 years later?! Let's head to another part of history:

ANCIENT GREEKS

Oils, perfumes, makeup, potions, powders and hair dyes were used almost universally in Ancient Greece. Many people made their own skincare from local, natural ingredients like fresh berries and milk. The Ancient Greeks also used olives and olive oil as exfoliants and moisturizers. Lastly, honey along with milk and yogurt were used as anti-aging preparations, in a similar way to the Ancient Egyptians.

However, the Ancient Greeks tended to just see their skin as a casing, or a vessel. However, the term *derma* (as in the words dermal, dermatology, dermatologist) comes from the Ancient Greek language and was originally used to mean the skin of a vegetable or animal. They did, however, view skin problems as outward representations of internal imbalance. It was Greek medical pioneer Galen who recognized the skin as an organ.

MEDIEVAL TIMES

Smooth, white skin was highly regarded in Europe in medieval times. Many women used herbal remedies to promote fair skin and diminish pimples. Ointments using animal fats were used. Aloe vera, rosemary, and cucumbers were used to cleanse the skin. Seeds, leaves, and flowers were also mixed with honey to create face masks, and vinegar was used as an astringent.

RENAISSANCE

Women in the Renaissance period used silver mercury, lead, and chalk to color their faces and make it appear whiter. This was extremely hazardous and led to widespread illness and death for the women using these products. Most of the skin care practices were the same as the medieval period, and women primarily relied on herbs and honey to cleanse and rejuvenate their skin. Some other skin care remedies included using broom stalks to cleanse the skin and oatmeal boiled in vinegar to treat pimples. Bread soaked in rose water was also used to soothe puffy eyes.

THE BAROQUE ERA

During the Baroque Era, women believed in saunas and sweat cleansing. Milk baths were also used for smoother, clearer skin. Makeup during this time was intended to look like paint, and heavy makeup was considered more respectable (again, similar to trends from the last 50 years at least). Rouge was very popular, and in the 1780s, French women used two million pots of rouge per year. Women's lips were reddened with distilled alcohol or vinegar.

1800'S

Exercise, cleanliness, and skincare were a big deal in the 1800's. Zinc oxide was used to lighten skin, but often caused allergic reactions. Hygiene products became easier to get hold of and harsh cleansers were often used. Egg yolks, honey and oatmeal were often also used to soften the skin and help diminish blemishes. Lemon juice was also used to naturally bleach the skin a few shades lighter (more on modern skin bleaching later). Chapstick, Vaseline and baby powder were invented, all of which were used in skincare regimens at this time.

Dermatology began to be recognized as a medical speciality of its own around the 18th or 19th century.

1900'S

The 1900's were an explosion in terms of accessible skincare for women. Carmex was invented in the 1930's, with the 1940's bringing us sunscreen and the launch of Estee Lauder. The 1950's brought us Clearasil, Ponds, Oil of Olay and Clinique all launched too. Trends came and went. The 1980's saw a rise in interest in natural skincare products. Then in the early 2000's the FDA approved Botox for frown lines on the face - it's thought that millions of the frown-freezing injections now take place every year.

Let's park the general history lesson here and move on to something that's close to my heart, and hopefully yours too.

A BRIEF HISTORY OF THE BLACK SKINCARE AND BEAUTY INDUSTRY

We're going to focus on the black beauty industry over the last 100 or so years. This is mainly going to be about the US and Canada as it's not intended to be a history book all about the roots of the beauty industry, but more to give you a flavor of how and why we are where we are.

Let's talk about some of the founders of the black beauty industry in the US first and foremost:

Madam CJ Walker

One of the most well-known black beauty entrepreneurs in the US was Sarah Breedlove, also known as CJ Walker. In 1905 she became the first Black American woman to become a self-made millionaire, all through her namesake cosmetic line and hair products. Netflix made a movie inspired by her life called Self-Made if you want to check that out.

Anthony Overton

In 1891, entrepreneur Anthony Overton opened Overton Hygienic Manufacturing, which sold cosmetics, perfumes, hair products and toiletries (some of which were tailored for use with black skin like the High-Brown Face Powder created to stop black women from experiencing ashiness with white face powders). This was one of the first cosmetics companies in the US to specifically create cosmetics for black women. His company exported around the world and allowed him to even establish his own bank and insurance company.

Annie Malone

Annie Malone struggled with illness and loss in her life, using this free time to experiment with hair and beauty. In 1902 she opened her first store and sold a line she called Poro Skin and Hair, including cold creams and vanishing creams to be used under powder. This made her the first commercially available black skincare founder and one of the first black millionaires in the US.

Poro Skin and Hair was extremely popular - and part of her success was that she was a black woman, designing and producing products for other black women. Other brands who did not have black founders sold unsafe products, gave poor advice and marketed their products by explaining - to black women - how lighter skin was more desirable.

Marjorie Joyner

Marjorie had previously owned her own salon, with her experience in the industry leading to the creation of a permanent hair wave machine. She filed a patent for this machine in 1928 then went on to co-found the United Beauty School Owners and Teachers Association and associated sorority and fraternity. These still exist today to uplift educational and economic standards within the beauty industry.

John H. Johnson

John was a publisher who had commercial publishing ventures aimed at the black community. He also owned Supreme Beauty Products and Fashion Fair Cosmetics, the largest black-owned cosmetics company in the world at the time. Fashion Fair had been created specifically for women of color. They went on to manufacture skincare, fragrance and hair care products.

Kashmir Chemical Co.

In 1918, Kashmir Chemical Co formed (made up of black investors) and debuted a hair and skincare line called Nile

Queen. They had unique access to black media outlets and celebrities and were able to grow into an extremely popular black beauty brand. Less than 10 years later, the company was hit with a lawsuit from a competitor as the name Kashmir was similar to one of their own product lines. Although they won the lawsuit, the business didn't recover from the financial strain and the business was dissolved.

Rose Meta Morgan

Rose opened a salon in 1945 in New York, to offer hair and skin care services for black women. The salon went on to sell products and made more than $3 million in sales within a few years of opening. Rose went on to move into banking and helped set up Freedom National bank, a black-owned commercial bank in New York.

WHAT DOES THIS MEAN FOR THE BLACK SKINCARE AND BEAUTY INDUSTRY TODAY?

So there we have it, a brief history of the beauty industry over time. Along with the impact of black entrepreneurs on the industry.

The black community has needed (and have been using) products specifically to meet the needs of their skin and hair for hundreds of years, and thousands more in history.

Some of the ideas behind brands that we've outlined earlier, the issues along the way and the attitudes that these businesses have been met with sound surprisingly familiar.

Over one hundred years later and it still feels like there's a lack of representation, understanding and familiarity of the needs of black skin and hair. It's often an afterthought, or included as something that feels inauthentic.

Things are improving, with a raft of new black beauty founders and more inclusive training but there are still times where black skin is something to be concerned about when it comes to skin treatments and products.

SKIN THEOLOGIAN'S TIP

I've worked with many fantastic beauty and skincare brands over the years. With brands that aren't representative - particularly at a decision making level - of their customer, it can lead to a lack of understanding of the needs and issues that customers, such as those with darker skin tones, face. This can sometimes mean that there's a lack of perspective in product development, shade ranges and imagery.

It may surprise you to discover that some of the hair and beauty brands that you know, love and think of as unequivocally "black" don't have black founders, or have no-one at a senior level who reflects their target audience, or are overwhelmingly staffed by people who aren't black and don't understand the consumer need from within.

I'm absolutely not saying that people can't learn, and that a product is better or worse because it was developed by a person of a certain skin color. However it goes back to the age-old problem of products being developed and marketed to make money from black consumers, without that money supporting the black community to use their knowledge, grow and thrive.

If understanding how brands represent people like you and your experiences is important to you (hint: it should be), there are lots of online resources that outline who owns which brands, their staffing ratios and who their target audiences are.

It's important to support the right, inclusive brands, whoever founded them. Many of the newer brands like Fenty, Humanrace, Melyon and many more have inclusivity - of everyone - at their core and we should absolutely embrace that change.

SKIN IN THE HERE AND NOW

Let's move away from history and move on to science.

We talked a little about the structure of the skin earlier and some of the common conditions, but let's continue on with the theme of going a little deeper and really get into some detail about the anatomy of the human skin - all skin types.

Human skin is the covering of the body that provides protection and receives signals from the external environment. It consists of three layers - the epidermis, stratum corneum and the dermis. It's also supported by the subcutis, a layer of fat beneath the dermis that supplies nutrients and provides cushioning.

Skin is its own little ecosystem, filled with bacteria and microorganisms that work together in harmony to protect your skin (and the rest of your body). It's a delicate balance that can be thrown out of whack by our lifestyle, the products we use, the food we eat and even things like whether we have pets and how much we touch our face.

Your skin changes throughout your life. Infants usually have dry, soft skin that's free of blemishes and wrinkles. As you get older, sun exposure, genetics and lifestyle have an impact on your skin. This is where things like age spots, wrinkles and fine lines come into play.

Skin is extremely strong and pliable, the layers working together to complement one another. There are also countless nerve endings throughout the skin that help us to sense and feel our environment.

SKIN THEOLOGIAN'S TIP

This isn't a book about hair, but when you talk about the skin on the face, we often forget about our scalp. We rarely see it, but it's an extension of the skin on our face and isn't always treated that way. It ages, it can be dry or oily, it can struggle with skin conditions.

Scalp care is essential for healthy hair and skin - so don't forget about yours! Get into good routines, and think about your scalp the way you would your skin.

THE SURFACE OF YOUR SKIN

The surface of your skin is covered in pores, sweat glands and hair follicles. They're in unique patterns, just like fingerprints and are established before birth. Pores are a completely normal part of (the) skin. Everyone has them.

For some people, especially oilier or more mature skin, pores can be more visible or look larger. Again, this is normal and relates to how your skin is naturally made. Pores can also become clogged with dead skin and sebum, causing blackheads or pimples. Unfortunately, these clogs can stretch out your pores, making them appear larger for good.

MYTHBUSTING WITH THE SKIN THEOLOGIAN

MYTH: "You can shrink, open and close your pores."

TRUTH: You're not going to like this...pores don't actually have any muscle structure to them so they can't open or close. Your pore is just there, doing it's thing at all times of the day.

The other thing to be aware of is that once a pore is enlarged and stretched out, it's usually now that size for good. Sometimes, if a pore has been clogged and inflamed, it looks way smaller once it's unclogged which could be where this myth comes from. Some products can temporarily have a slight effect.

HOW DOES SKIN CHANGE AS A RESULT OF OUR ENVIRONMENT?

As we've mentioned previously, skin is affected by lifestyle, genetics and UV rays from the sun. The natural aging process - that happens to us *all* - also plays a part. We're obsessed with looking younger and chasing that fountain of youth. Unfortunately, it doesn't exist!

There are ways you can take care of your skin to keep it looking youthful for longer, but aging is something that happens while the years roll by. We'll talk a little more about that later on.

The other thing to be aware of is how your skin can change throughout the year, especially if you live in a climate where the seasons really do change. Cold weather, the sun, humidity, wind and rain all affect our skin - stay conscious of how the changing seasons affect your skin so you can be aware of how you need to change up your routine.

KEY TAKEAWAYS

- Skincare isn't a new concept, however much the latest new product launch might try and convince us of that fact.
- Black skincare and beauty brands have existed for a long time, but continue to face some of the same challenges even 100+ years later.
- Your skin is a finely-tuned balancing act that's working to protect your body, and changes throughout your life.

*If you're enjoying this book so far, we'd love to know your thoughts. Drop us your review on Audible and on Amazon. Under the review section of The No Compromise Black Skin Care Guide: The Truth About Caring For Darker Skin. http://amazon.com/review/create-review/asin=B0979PBM7.

4

PRIMARY AND COMMON CONCERNS WITH BLACK SKIN

In this chapter, you'll learn about:

- Some of the key concerns facing black and darker skin tones
- How to handle some of these common concerns
- Taking care of your body

As I've mentioned throughout this book, there are some skin conditions, concerns and talking points that are unique to black and darker skin. Some are prevalent throughout all skin types and tones, but more common in black skin.

I've touched on these conditions throughout the book but let's go deeper and talk about why they're more prevalent in darker skin, what you need to know about them and what steps to take to deal with these concerns.

HYPERPIGMENTATION, DARK SPOTS AND DISCOLORATION

This was the big issue that almost every skin professional I asked said was the main concern that their clients with black or darker skin presented. It's something I get asked about frequently. It's something my clients worry about and in general that people want solutions for as they want an even skin tone.

Hyperpigmentation is the overproduction of melanin in the skin following sun damage, acne or a skin wound. It's basically the skin overcompensating during the healing process by producing so much melanin that it's visibly darker on the skin.

Post-Inflammatory Pigmentation (PIH) can happen after skin is inflamed, usually due to conditions like eczema, ingrown hairs, bites or acne. It can affect the top layer of the skin and even the further layer underneath. This is one of the reasons that you need to try and avoid inflammation if you have black or darker skin.

Chemical peeling and laser treatments can be used for more extensive hyperpigmentation along with topical treatments. It's best to seek guidance from a professional on this as there are some things you need to be aware of when it comes to these treatments.

Melasma is another skin disorder that leads to discoloration. It's where patches of pigment appear at high points of the face (cheeks, bridge of the nose, upper lip and forehead). It's usually genetic and related to sun exposure and hormones. It's harder to treat than some other types of discoloration so prevention is your best bet.

SKIN THEOLOGIAN'S TIP

It's completely normal to have different skin tones on your face - to the point where you may use different shades of makeup to "correct" it or balance it out. Hyperpigmentation is normal and is something that many people experience. It isn't just you.

It's also normal for your body and face to be different shades, whatever your skin tone or complexion. No-one's skin is one completely matching shade all over.

As we mentioned, because of hyperpigmentation, there are a few things to consider when you have black skin and are thinking about treatments:

Laser treatments

Be careful when it comes to laser treatments, whether that's hair removal or for skin rejuvenation purposes.

At one end of the spectrum, it may be ineffective - hair removal with laser sometimes doesn't work with darker skin tones as the laser works by picking out the darker pigment of hairs, so works best with dark hair and light skin. Some are better than others so do your research and choose your professional wisely.

Some lasers aren't good for black and darker skin tones, and can contribute to hyperpigmentation. There are other laser treatments that can be used safely on darker skin. Speak to your dermatologist or skin professional about this - ideally you want to have a skilled, certified dermatologist who is experienced in using laser devices on dark skin to carry out your treatment.

Chemical peels and acid treatments

The premise of these types of treatment is that they use chemicals to peel the skin. These treatments can sometimes be too aggressive for darker skin tones and can cause more problems with PIH when used incorrectly.

It's best to go easy on this and again, work with an experienced and trained professional to address these issues. You want the person using acids on your skin to be confident and clear on what they're doing, whatever your skin tone.

Facials

Facials can be an amazing way to destress, relax, deal with skincare concerns and get some much-needed me-time. However, it's not all plain sailing when it comes to hyperpigmentation. Proceed with caution when it comes to things like extractions - a heavy handed approach (even with the best intentions) from your facialist can lead to, yep you guessed it, scarring and PIH.

I'm definitely not saying a facial is something to be avoided. I carry out hundreds of them every year - honestly, thousands over the course of my career - to clients of all skin tones. They love them and their skin really does benefit. But you need someone who's experienced with black skin, which is why I want professionals to have this experience and feel confident.

Skin Bleaching

Skin bleaching has, unfortunately, been part of the black community for a long time. It has roots in many different historical elements. From women who saw extremely pale skin as the height of beauty in the 1800's, from the media who have championed lighter skin as the only route to beauty and even in colonialism across the world.

Colorism within our own communities, families and social circle still exists, as does the false narrative that lighter skin is "better" across the media. The issue is a complex one rooted in history as well as the here and now, and happens all over the world.

It's estimated that across the world women of color are spending more than $8 billion on bleaching creams every year. This is despite these products being banned in many countries, and despite the fact that many of them include hazardous chemicals such as mercury, bleaching agents and steroids.

It's popular in many African countries, the Caribbean, India and the Middle East - as well as countries such as the US, Canada and the UK. Bleaching creams in these countries are often marketed as being used to "erase blemishes" and "age spots", which they can be used for but more often than not are used for wider skin-bleaching.

The other issue comes when people try and make their own concoctions to lighten their skin - there have been reports of people applying dangerous ingredients such as car battery acid, cloth bleaching agents and home detergents to their skin in a bid to lighten it.

It goes without saying that this is extremely dangerous, toxic, bad for health and should never, ever, ever be done.

Rather than point fingers at individuals, it's the societal pressure and low self-esteem that's forced on women with darker skin tones that is to blame, and the likely reason why many women choose to bleach their skin.

There is more education going on around bleaching creams - Johnson & Johnson no longer sell a number of products that were marketed this way, and L'Oreal have pledge to remove wording like "light", "white" and "fair" from the products they sell this way but will continue to sell them, at the time of writing.

The fact of the matter is that skin bleaching comes with many, many risks and is so bad for your beautiful, dark skin. It can cause rashes, discoloration and scarring as well as affect your skin's natural resistance to infection.

It will make your skin more sensitive to the sun and could leave you at risk of developing serious skin issues, such as skin cancer.

It's also bad for your health away from "just" your skin. The World Health Organization has said that skin bleaching can cause liver and kidney damage, neurological problems, cancer, and stillbirths in pregnant women. They've also said that the issue of skin bleaching should be prioritized as a public health concern.

As a side note, large-scale skin bleaching - especially on darker skin tones - often leaves the skin with an unnatural, dull gray tone that's a million miles away from the rich tones that come with darker, melanin-rich skin. Skin is not meant to be a dull, one-dimensional gray tone.

Skin bleaching "treatments" (I hate to even call it a treatment, as it's essentially destroying your skin) or methods tend to work in the following ways:

- Inhibiting the activity of an enzyme called Tyrosinase. This enzyme is what the body converts into melanin so by holding it back the idea is that it holds back melanin production too.
- Preventing melanin from being deposited onto the skin. Some processes stop melanin from getting from

your body to the surface of your skin. Over time the melanin is not replaced.
- Destruction of melanin and melanocytes to stop melanin production.

I'll pause for a moment. Does any of the above actually sound good to you? Or like it's something that's good for your health?

In case you're not already convinced, let's look at some of the common ingredients that are used in skin bleaching and why they're bad news.

Hydroquinone

A frequently-used bleaching agent that's banned across the world - is often responsible for that gray tone. It can also cause premature aging and weakening of your skin. In the longer term, widespread use can cause problems with your nervous system and liver.

Mercury

Products that contain mercury to lighten your skin are toxic. That's it. They're completely toxic. And I don't mean that in the way the beauty industry sometimes talks about "toxins" without really meaning anything. Mercury is a toxic element that will accumulate in your body and cause damage to your essential organs like your kidney, liver and brain. Not worth it. Don't do it.

Steroids

Creams that incorporate steroids can cause skin thinning, stretch marks, bruising easily and broken veins. Over time and longer-term use (especially across your entire body) can cause problems with blood pressure, diabetes, osteoporosis and weight gain.

There are also tablets and injections that are said to lighten skin. These interfere with your body's natural melanin production. In some forms, there's no scientific evidence that it even works to lighten skin. There is however, scientific evidence that these methods can cause severe skin rashes, kidney and thyroid disease.

So, to recap here's why skin bleaching should be avoided at all costs:

- You don't need to do it. Skin of all tones is beautiful, including yours.
- It can come with serious risks to your health - including your kidneys, liver, brain and other organs.
- It's bad for your skin and can cause irritation, sun sensitivity and rashes.
- It can cause premature aging of the skin.
- Weakens your skin.
- It can cause discoloration of your skin.
- Can leave an unnatural gray tone across your whole skin.

SKIN THEOLOGIAN'S TIP

Black skin is beautiful. Say no to bleaching.

That's it, that's my tip in relation to skin bleaching.

You should never, ever use bleaching agents on your skin in the long term or over large portions of your face and/or body (tiny areas of dark spots, maybe, as directed and with extreme caution in very specific cases and under professional guidance).

You don't need to bleach your skin, change your skin color or aspire to be lighter. It's not you. You are truly beautiful and should be proud of your beautiful melanin and the cultural history, heritage and love that made it.

If you feel like your darker skin "isn't good enough" (spoiler alert: your skin is far more than "good enough") take the time to look at where that perception is coming from. Curate your social media feeds to show more black women with skin just like yours, move conversations with friends and family away from lighter skin, celebrate your melanin and take the time to educate yourself on the cultural issues around darker skin and skin bleaching.

You don't need to do it. Risking your health to be a few shades lighter isn't worth it and isn't necessary.

Pseudo Folliculitis

(aka razor bumps, razor burn or ingrown hairs)

This is a common one for black men, but can obviously affect women too. Because of the texture and curl pattern of black hair, when facial hair is cut with a razor it can curl back on itself and grow into the skin. This isn't exclusive to black and darker skin but is more of a problem due to those curls.

This ingrown hair can be painful and can cause inflammation, which can then lead to - fanfare please - hyperpigmentation and/or infection.

Using the right razor is key for prevention. Taking steps to avoid ingrown hairs is usually easier than dealing with the consequences, and less painful for your skin. There are single blade razors that have been made especially with curly hair in mind. Regular exfoliation and moisturizing can also help to reduce the number of ingrown hairs (and to tackle any PIH you may be experiencing as a result).

Having the correct shaving technique (there are lots of tutorials out there - personal tip: shave in the direction of hair growth, not against it.) prepping your skin properly and using the right products when shaving can all help with the process too. There are also other hair removal products that are available, such as hair removal powder.

Women can also be affected by this condition on their face too, as well as on areas where they remove hair like legs or their bikini line.It might be a better option to wax, but everyone has their own preferences.

Keloid Scarring

This is more common in darker skin tones, though there isn't nearly enough research into keloids and the reasons why they occur. If others in your family get keloids then it's more likely that you will too. Around 10% of the entire population (of all skin types and tones) experience keloid scarring.

A keloid is extreme scarring that forms during the healing process, but goes over the edges of the original wound. They're usually thick, fleshy and raised.

Caused by collagen overproduction, they develop after injury or trauma to the skin. This can be anything from acne, piercings, surgery, vaccination, blisters and skin injuries. They can develop months or years after the trauma and tend to carry on growing, eventually stopping.

They aren't always painful, but they can cause discomfort and itchiness. Depending on where they are (for example an area over a joint or where skin is "tight") they can be uncomfortable. Many people find their keloids unsightly from a cosmetic point of view and seek treatment on this basis, as well as discomfort.

If you know you're predisposed to keloids, prevention is the best option. If you really struggle with keloid scarring then it might be that you avoid piercings, tattoos and some cosmetic procedures that involve cutting or injecting into the skin.

Where keloids are already present, they can be surgically removed but this can obviously come with a risk of further scarring, pigmentation changes and the return of the scarring. There are also some topical treatments and non-surgical interventions like treatment with Botulinum toxin or cryotherapy.

This is one to discuss with your doctor as there may be less-invasive treatments to try before surgery is on the cards.

Keloids are sometimes confused with hypertrophic scars - they're flat, usually caused by injuries and can go away on their own.

Dry/Ashy Skin on your Body

Sometimes discussion around skincare is limited to just talking about the face. Whilst your face (along with your hands and neck) are usually the most visible part of your skin - as well as the part that gets the most exposure to the sun and your environment - don't forget it covers your whole body too!

With black and darker skin, dry skin can look gray and ashy. It may also feel rough or bumpy and show thin, cracked lines - it can even peel, flake or bleed in extreme cases. You can have oily skin and still have dry patches. Dry skin is most common on areas like the knees, elbows and feet but can appear anywhere on the body.

Dry skin is different - and looks different - to skin conditions like eczema, dermatitis and psoriasis. These conditions usually need medical intervention, whereas dry skin can be managed as part of a normal skincare routine.

Cold, harsh weather and dry air can cause dry skin, as can showers and baths that are too hot. Some products that contain harsh chemicals that strip your skin of its natural moisture can also lead to dry skin.

Here's how to avoid - and deal with - ashy skin:

- If hot showers and baths are your thing, it's time to cool it down. Lukewarm water and limiting the amount of time you spend in the water can be beneficial.
- Change your products to moisturizing, nourishing ones rather than stripping your skin of its natural moisture. Products for sensitive skin are usually more gentle.
- Moisturize your skin daily. Do it right after a bath or a shower, before you go outside.
- Petroleum jelly, where it has been properly used to lock in moisture, can block the skin as a barrier. The downside is that it can be sticky or greasy, so this is

one to use when you don't need to go anywhere and when it won't ruin your clothes! For deep moisture locking treatments, consider using therapeutic ingredients rather than mineral oil or petroleum jelly.
- Humidifiers at home can help to stop dry air (especially if you're running the heat at home during winter).
- Up your water intake to prevent dehydration. This obviously has other health benefits for your body as well as skin and hair.

KEY TAKEAWAYS

- The risk of hyperpigmentation is real, and it's a concern for people with darker or black skin. Prevention is best where possible.
- Always consult a professional if you're not sure, or need specific help or advice on how to deal with common conditions.
- Skin bleaching is extremely dangerous for your skin (and completely unnecessary).
- Keloid scarring is best prevented as the treatment of them can be challenging.
- The skin on your body needs care, as well as your face. Start a simple routine and banish ashiness.

5

LET'S LEVEL-UP ON INGREDIENTS

*I*n this chapter, you'll learn about:

- Building a skincare routine
- The ingredients that your skin needs
- What ingredients do for your skin

Sometimes when it comes to skincare it can feel like you need to throw on a lab coat and think back to your science class. Quite often, nothing seems to be as straightforward as it should be.

The beauty industry is full of acronyms, product names written in Latin, pseudo-science, marketing buzzwords and some ingredients that are just straight up bad for your skin.

However, the beauty industry is also filled with amazing, effective products that have been developed by the best cosmetic scientists to really make a difference to your skin.

Let's talk about some of the ingredients that are commonly used in skincare products for darker skins and how to start building a simple skincare routine.

BUILDING YOUR SKINCARE ROUTINE

First things first - a different daytime and nighttime skincare routine is essential. If you've worn makeup, been exposed to pollution or been sweating through the day then this all needs to be removed with something a little more heavy duty than what you'd use in your morning routine.

Second thing, yes you should wash your face when you wake up. You still sweat when you're asleep and your skin continues to produce oils overnight, which can lead to blocked pores if not removed from your face.

I like to say that the skin is in defence mode throughout the day and repair mode at night. Just because you're sleeping, it doesn't mean your skin is! When we're asleep, our skin is highly active repairing and renewing itself.

SKIN THEOLOGIAN'S TIP

Wash and change your pillow cases regularly. You might be wondering what that has to do with your skin, right? Everything. You put your face on your pillow every night (that same face that's sweating and producing oil every night) then do it all over again the next bedtime. This can lead to clogged pores.

Even better, invest in a pure silk pillowcase (but still wash it regularly) as they can be more beneficial for skin and hair.

DAYTIME SKINCARE ROUTINE

Hop out of bed and straight into your morning routine. Here are the steps that you should take for your morning routine:

1. **Cleanse** - use a gentle cleanser to remove oil-based debris first of all. A second cleanse (it can be with the same cleanser) then removes water-based impurities from the skin's surface.
2. **Tone** - some people skip this step but if you have a toner that you like, then you should definitely be using it.

3. **Serum** - a vitamin C serum can be great to help prevent sun and pollution damage.
4. **Eye Cream** - dab an eye cream on (gently) to your delicate eye area.
5. **Moisturizer** - this keeps your skin hydrated and helps to strengthen your skin's natural barrier. For daytime routines, use a lighter moisturizer.
6. **Sunscreen** - protect your skin with a good quality sunscreen.

Then continue with the rest of your morning routine (including makeup if you wear it) to head out and start your day.

NIGHTTIME ROUTINE

Get ready for bed and a night of beauty sleep with this easy evening routine:

1. **Cleanse** - use a gentle cleanser to remove dirt/makeup and oil from the skin's surface. You might want to try an oil based cleanser, or double-cleansing to make sure you've removed your make up and cleaned your skin.
2. **Tone** - as above, if you use it (*and you should*) then now's the time.
3. **Serum** - a vitamin A retinol is better used at night. (Retinol helps to stimulate collagen and increases cell

turnover, while the skin is in repair mode at night. Also, Vitamin A can be sun sensitizing in the daytime (which can leave pigmentation…a major concern for darker skin), so it is ideal for night-time use.

4. **Eye Cream** - dab an eye cream on (gently) to your delicate eye area.
5. **Acne or zit treatments** - if this is something you experience, then the night is a good time for these topical treatments to work their magic. (use as directed in the product directions. I advise a targeted treatment, a little, goes a long way.
6. **Moisturizer** - this keeps your skin hydrated and helps to strengthen your skin's natural barrier. You can go a little heavier and nourishing at night. (As we lose moisture naturally while we sleep. Consider a moisturizer with great levels of Hyaluronic Acid.)
7. **Face Oil** - add an extra boost of moisture at night to hydrate and soften the skin. (Don't worry, oil does not mean bad, even if you are oily! There are healthy oils that help to control bad oils in our skin. Just like there are healthy fats in our diet that help us to lose bad fats in our body.)

MYTHBUSTING WITH THE SKIN THEOLOGIAN

MYTH: "Oily skin should steer clear of using oils."

TRUTH: Not true. Oils can actually be beneficial for oily skin and can actually help to stop your skin overproducing oil, as it has everything it needs. If you have oily skin then avoid oils that are known to clog pores like coconut oil and mineral oil on your face.

SOME EXTRA INFO FOR YOUR ROUTINE

In addition to your daily routine, there are also some weekly skincare treats you might want to incorporate into your overall skincare routine:

- **Exfoliation** - using a chemical (or physical, if that's your thing) exfoliator to remove dead skin cells and reveal the younger-looking, renewed and refreshed skin underneath. Over exfoliating can be really bad for your skin so don't overdo it as your skin needs time to replenish itself.
- **Face masks/treatments** - use a treatment that's suitable for your skin type and any conditions once a week (or however often the manufacturer instructs).

- **Check your face over** - for any new signs of aging, hyperpigmentation or skin issues (such as abnormal growths). It's better to be vigilant when it comes to aging and damage.

SKIN THEOLOGIAN'S TIP

Change up your routine with the seasons. If it's snowing outside, your skin will have different needs than when it's the hottest point of summer.

Try and keep track of how your skin behaves and what it needs when the weather changes.

Sometimes, you'll just want to change your routine, or your skin will let you know when it's time to try something new! Work with the condition of your skin first of all.

COMMONLY USED SKINCARE INGREDIENTS

I've pulled together a quick reference for some of the more common ingredients that are used in skincare. It's sometimes a little bit of trial and error to find out which are right for you (as skincare is often so personal), but getting the right ones can make a phenomenal difference to your skin:

Acids

If you're new to skincare, you might be thinking "is putting acid on your skin a good idea?" The answer is that it depends on your skin and the acid you're looking to use. Acids are used for lots of different things, here's a quick round up

Glycolic acid

An AHA exfoliant with antioxidant and anti-inflammatory purposes. It loosens the bond between dead and living skin cells, causing them to shed and reveal underlying, fresh skin. Glycolic acid is used for anti-aging, reducing age spots, acne and scarring, hyperpigmentation, melasma and oily skin.

Lactic Acid

Made from milk, this acid is used to tackle signs of aging, fine lines and wrinkles through exfoliation to encourage shedding. On dark skin, this also gently lifts dullness from the complexion.

Mandelic Acid

This is a mild acid made from almonds. It's also an exfoliant that works really well on oily or acne-prone skin, and to treat hyperpigmentation. It reduces oil without drying the skin out.

Salicylic Acid

Derived from Willow Bark (you'll sometimes see it referred to as 'Willow Bark Extract' on ingredients), this acid has an anti-inflammatory effect to calm breakouts. (It also is wonderfully, anti-bacterial). Best for oily or acne-prone skin types it can penetrate deep into the pores and break down dead skin cells to avoid blocked pores. I call it the 'triple threat acid': anti-inflammatory, anti-bacterial and oil-loving.

Azelaic Acid

Made from grains like barley, rye and wheat, this is a great one to use against acne. It's also used to treat hyperpigmentation and dark marks, as well as helping skin cells to shed. It has some antibacterial properties too.

Hyaluronic Acid

This acid is made naturally in the body and helps skin to retain water (also known as a humectant), but is also lost as we age which can lead to dry skin and wrinkles. Dehydrated or dry darker skin tends to look dull or gray, and hyaluronic acid can help with this. Hyaluronic acid can also be used as a dermal filler to plump up lines and wrinkles. It has the wonderful ability to hold one thousand times its own weight in moisture. So it's a great way to prevent water loss in the skin.

Antioxidants

Antioxidants protect the skin from free radical damage. They delay signs of ageing and prevent inflammation. Their anti-inflammatory response protects the skin against sun damage and photoaging, preventing sunburn, dark spots and uneven skin tone.

One of the best known antioxidants is vitamin C. It helps wound healing, boosting collagen production, brightening dark spots. Hence, it protects from UV damage and pollution. It helps correct dark spots and prevent future skin damage and discoloration.

Vitamins

Your skin needs vitamins and nutrients to thrive. You can get these from a balanced diet, supplements and through applying to your skin topically.

Here's a quick guide to which vitamin does what for your skin:

Vitamin A - used for conditions like acne and psoriasis but also hyperpigmentation. It speeds up cell turnover to reveal clearer, fresher skin. Retinoids are derived from vitamin A and can help with collagen production and wrinkle reduction.

Vitamin C - great for dark skin as it helps with collagen production, skin protection from UV rays and can help to reduce hyperpigmentation as well as repairing damaged skin. Look for stabilized vitamin C, as it is also one of the hardest vitamins to stabilize.

Vitamin D - we get this from the sun and it's great for healthy bones and skin, Without it skin will appear thinner. Darker skin tones need more Vitamin D as the natural melanin in the skin stops as much being absorbed.

Vitamin B3 - plays a role in your skin's natural barrier through reducing water loss, increasing ceramides and helping with regeneration of cells.

Vitamin B5 - essential for normal functioning of the epidermis. It has anti-inflammatory and moisturizing effects on the skin and this helps to reduce water loss and improve the hydration of the epidermis to help the skin maintain suppleness and elasticity.

> **SKIN THEOLOGIAN'S TIP**
>
> Not all vitamin ingredients are created equally. Look for stabilized formulation-grades that secure the function of these amazing active ingredients.
>
> There are different qualities of vitamins used in products. This is the same across most ingredients, but the difference with vitamins is that they need to use a stable formulation to actually work on the skin.
>
> Even product packaging, storage conditions and ingredients combinations can make a difference to product effectiveness. Brands don't always take this into account when making products, so you need to.
>
> If your product is changing color, separating or smells different, then this could be a sign of instability. Also, products have a shelf-life - keep an eye on it!

Ceramides

Ceramides are responsible for keeping skin plump and smooth. They naturally appear in the skin, maintaining moisture levels and strengthen barrier function but come in lots of different forms.

Squalane

This occurs naturally and is one of the most common lipids in the skin. It starts to reduce by the age of 30 which can be when dry skin kicks in. Usually in oil format, it's more stable than other types of oil and doesn't feel greasy. It's a great ingredient for acne-prone skin.

Allantoin

Promotes a healthy skin barrier by replenishing moisture content in the skin, enhancing its natural exfoliation process, reducing irritation and improving smoothness.

mBeta-Glucan

mBeta Glucan has been recognised for its immunomodulatory, antifungal and antiviral activities. They are higher than those of any other glucan complex carbohydrate.

To reduce the appearance of existing dark spots, people can use a specialized product. These include ingredients such as:

- Retinoids: Over-the-counter topical differin and prescription-based products such as tretinoin can be helpful.
- Hydroquinone: Products containing hydroquinone stop the production of excess melanin, which causes dark spots. However this should be used with caution

as it can be damaging to the skin with improper use, and has been banned in some countries. Ask your medical professional for guidance on whether hydroquinone is right for you. There are other options available that may be lower risk.
- Kojic acid: This is another skin lightener that can reduce dark spots, but it may be less effective.
- Vitamin C: Some researchTrusted Source suggests that vitamin C, an antioxidant, can reduce hyperpigmentation, protect against sun damage, and increase collagen levels. However, vitamin C has a poor ability to penetrate the skin, so more research into its effectiveness for these purposes is necessary.

Use of these products — particularly hydroquinone and kojic acid — with caution, as overuse could irritate the skin.

It is important to not use hydroquinone for extended periods of time. Aim to take a break after 3 months of continuous use. After long periods of use, hydroquinone can result in darkening of the skin. This is part of a condition called exogenous ochronosis.

Dermatologists may recommend a combination product that combines multiple products into one that people can use on their skin.

INGREDIENTS BLACK SKIN SHOULD AVOID

There are some products that just aren't right for darker skins as they can cause further issues. Here's some to sense check (or patch test) before you use:

- **Glycolic acid** - this (in higher concentrations) can cause post inflammatory hyperpigmentation in skin of colour
- **Alpha lipoic acid** - this powerful antioxidant can feel oily and can burn
- **Hydroquinone** - for skin of color, it can lead to contact dermatitis and hyperpigmentation.

Inflammation

We've talked about hyperpigmentation quite a bit already but it's important and one of the biggest skin concerns for black skin. What we need to talk about alongside is inflammation, as this is the big cause of hyperpigmentation. Avoiding inflammation for your skin is an essential part of preventing hyperpigmentation, and as prevention is often easier than treatment that's the route to take.

Here are some of the common causes of inflammation in black skin:

- **Acne, zits and blemishes** - these can cause inflammation and scarring.
- **Products** - using the wrong products or products that irritate your skin can cause inflammation. Tread carefully and test out products first if you're worried, have sensitive skin or react to certain ingredients.
- **Skin infections** - these can cause pain and inflammation in your skin.
- **Wounds** - damage to your skin can cause inflammation, swelling and infections.
- **Ingrown hairs** - ingrown hairs can cause inflammation, pain and swelling in the skin which can lead to hyperpigmentation.
- **Improper skincare treatments** - inexperienced professionals can use the wrong products, treatments or treat black skin too roughly, leading to hyperpigmentation.
- **UV exposure** - this can lead to inflammation in the skin and can darken hyperpigmentation-affected patches of skin.

KEY TAKEAWAYS

- Building a skincare routine is essential whatever your skin type, complexion or skin concerns.

- It might take a little trial and error to get the right mix of ingredients for your skin, but you will get there and the results will be amazing!
- Not every ingredient out there is right for black skin
- Inflammation should be avoided

TREATMENT SOLUTIONS

In this chapter, you'll learn about:

- Treatment solutions
- Aging skin
- When to speak to a professional

There are lots of different skincare treatments out there. They range from treatments that improve the skin on a temporary basis at the surface through to aesthetic treatments that change your skin for a longer period, right through to invasive, surgical interventions.

TREATMENTS FOR BLACK SKIN

Here are some of the treatments that can be extremely effective for black skin - some of these are best carried out by a professional who understands your skin and its needs:

Facials

We've talked a little about facial treatments. They can be extremely beneficial for your skin, especially when they're tailored to your skin and carried out by someone who knows what they're doing.

Chemical Peels

Great for acne, scarring, texture and pigmentation but be aware of the ingredient's use and leave it in the hands of an experienced professional to avoid hyperpigmentation and scarring.

Laser Skin Treatments

Best with a professional and great for pigmentation, dark spots and tightening your skin.

Microdermabrasion

This deep exfoliation treatment can remove dead skin and reveal a renewed, refreshed complexion underneath. It's great for dull or aging skin and can really make a difference.

Microneedling (aka Collagen Induction Therapy, Skin Needling or Dermarolling)

This can be great for reducing texture, scarring, pigmentation, wrinkles and more. The treatment you receive from a professional will be more intensive than what you'll experience using at-home rollers. Go easy on this and seek advice.

ANTI-AGING AND BLACK SKIN

As I mentioned earlier in the book, the phrase "black don't crack" isn't strictly true. Whilst it is true that darker skin shows signs of aging later than other skin, and that the melanin in our skin does give some protection against the sun (not enough - remember your sunscreen!), it isn't the case that we'll look like we're in our 20's forever.

Everyone gets older, and over time, you will start to see typical signs of aging such as fine lines, wrinkles, crows feet, uneven tone, larger pores and age spots, sagging and hyperpigmentation. Your skin may start to feel drier as you age too, as natural collagen and hyaluronic acid production slows down as we get older.

Remember, aging skin can still be dry, dull, acne-prone, mature or congested. Your skin type won't magically completely change as you age, though it might be a little different to what you're used to.

Here are some treatments that you can try at home to help with signs of aging in black skin:

Exfoliate and remove peach fuzz

Best carried out by a professional, dermaplaning uses a flat blade that removes peach fuzz and dead skin for a thorough exfoliating treatment. This can help to reveal the new skin underneath and stop skin from looking dry and dull. There are at-home options that you can use - I'd recommend going for the best tool you can afford and being careful with it to keep your skin safe.

Dealing with age spots

There are lots of treatments out there that exfoliate and brighten the skin without using chemicals like hydroquinone. Look for products that contain licorice root, kojic acid, arbutin, vitamin C, niacinamide, willow bark extract and lactic acid to help lighten dark spots and signs of aging at home without the side effects.

Reduce the appearance of pores

Our skin loses elasticity as we age which can make pores look larger. Your skin also gets thicker as you age, which again makes pores look bigger. Sun exposure and sagging skin also play their part in making your pores look more visible.

Sticking to a cleansing routine, using face masks and a regular exfoliation routine can all help to reduce the appearance of your pores. You can't shrink them, or remove them but you can keep them in check.

Boost your moisture

Even oily skin can suffer with dehydration, dryness and dullness. Getting enough water - at all ages - is important, and so is the way you treat your skin. No overly harsh cleansers on aging skin and use moisturizer daily (moisturizers that contain hyaluronic acid or vitamin C are great for adding moisture back into aging skin) .

Face masks are also a good way to give a deeper hit of hydration into your skin. The results are temporary, and I'd always recommend using a face mask that's intended to be used as a face mask rather than whipping up your own in the kitchen just so you can be sure that it's been tested and the balance of ingredients is right.

It comes down to preference and skincare needs when deciding what masks to use.

Here's what masks are best to treat specific issues:

- Clay and charcoal masks are best for detoxifying and removing excess oil.
- Sheet masks are great to use for a temporary hydration boost to your skin and can cool and soothe.
- Enzyme masks are usually used for physical exfoliation and brightening.

- Warming (or self-heating) masks help to bring blood to the surface of your skin and support circulation. Plus they can feel great!
- Brightening masks can help with pigmentation and skin tone and are great for dry, dull skin.
- Sleep masks are usually used for hydration and left on overnight.

SKIN THEOLOGIAN'S TIP

Always check the ingredients out in any face mask you use and avoid applying to any damaged, injured or delicate skin. If any of these are the case then it's best to seek medical advice for your skin's sake.

Bubble masks can look cute, for example, but they have no additional benefits to your skin and the foaming agents in them can actually irritate your skin. Not. Worth. It.

There are also lots of aesthetic treatments that can help with anti-aging such as anti-wrinkle injections, dermal fillers and things like PDO threads. Many of these treatments are seen as "not being for black skin" but often this is due to a lack of information and education, a lack of representation and that old "black don't crack" messaging.

Always speak to a medical professional before undertaking these kinds of treatments, and make sure you get the best, unbiased advice for your skin. You may feel better speaking to a doctor or dermatologist who looks like you, or has significant experience in treating patients who do and the cultural and medical differences in treating patients with black or darker skin.

Don't be afraid to walk away or get some thinking time if you're not 100%. These things are often a medical treatment and should be treated as such - it shouldn't be about the hard sell.

WHEN TO SPEAK TO A PROFESSIONAL

There are some things that take experience, qualifications and certifications to handle. There are some treatments that you simply can't do yourself due to skills, equipment and needing an extra pair of hands.

If you need advice, have specific concerns for you or you just want some time for yourself where someone takes care of you then don't be afraid to speak to a professional.

Whether that's an esthetician or facialist, a medical professional or dermatologist, it can be a route to quicker or more effective results for your skin. The amount of times a client has said to me "I wish I'd come to see you sooner!"

Don't struggle by yourself if your at-home treatments aren't working for you. Skin professionals see everything all day long and know what the best route is for you. They can recommend products, treatments and even just give general advice to improve your skin. They're there to help you reach your skin goals.

KEY TAKEAWAYS

- There are some treatments that you can do at home that are extremely effective.
- Some treatments can just feel nice and be pampering. And that's fine!
- Prevention is best when it comes to anti-aging but even if you're seeing signs of aging it's not too late to take action.
- Don't be afraid to reach out to a professional if you have specific concerns.

THE SKIN THEOLOGIAN'S 10 COMMANDMENTS FOR BLACK SKIN

*J*ust as a little reminder, I've created some skincare commandments for black and darker skin tones. This is just a little fun from me as the Skin Theologian but the message behind them all is serious, so take heed as you take care of your skin.

1. Thou shalt wear sunscreen

Protect your skin from hyperpigmentation, signs of aging, skin cancer and fine lines - they'll appear eventually - by applying sunscreen regularly as part of your sunscreen. Yes you need it, and no your natural melanin doesn't protect you 100%. Find a sunscreen you like that doesn't leave a cast on your skin and *use it*.

2. Don't believe that "black don't crack."

It can crack. It might take a little longer than some other skin tones but signs of aging will appear on your skin as you get older.

3. Skin bleaching is blasphemy

It's bad for your skin, it's bad for your health and it looks unnatural (because it is). Black and darker skin is beautiful in all tones, you don't need the bleach.

4. Thou shall be aware of hyperpigmentation

It comes in different forms with different causes, and a lot of us are concerned about it. Be aware of it and what causes it and take care of your skin.

5. Building a routine should be part of your gospel

Find the right products and routine for your skin, and sticking to it consistently will really benefit your skin. It doesn't have to be complicated or expensive either.

6. Research is an essential part of honoring your skin

Understanding your skin, the products you use and the brands you like is important. A little bit of research goes a long way, so familiarize yourself with your skincare.

7. Thou shalt feel good in your skin

Looking good shouldn't feel bad. And you shouldn't feel bad about the way you look. We all want to present our best selves, and we all have little things we do that make us feel better. Confidence, holding your head high and feeling great in your skin is really important.

8. Thou shalt listen to your skin

If there's a big trend that everyone is talking about, or a product that worked wonders for your best friend, but *your* skin hates it. Listen to your skin. Every product isn't for everyone. Skin is different from person to person.

9. Some things are best left in the holy hands of a professional

Some self-care is perfect to do at home. Other things like getting a diagnosis for a skin condition, invasive treatments or ones that need a delicate, experienced touch are best left with a pro. Whether that's an esthetician or a medical professional like a dermatologist.

10. Your body is a temple

Getting the right nourishment, nutrition and enough water is important for healthy skin, hair and nails. It's also good for your body and wellbeing. Remember, skin isn't just on your face - you need to take care of your body too!

CONCLUSION

The main takeaway from this entire book is that there's still work to be done. We need to realise just how beautiful black and darker skin is - as individuals, in society and in the professional beauty industry.

There's an opportunity for real change and education within the beauty industry, to create an industry that includes everyone and that everyone can be proud of.

Self care and skin care go hand in hand. Don't let anyone tell you otherwise, or make excuses to stop you from reaching your skin goals.

I'm proud of my skin and I'm proud to be a skin professional in the industry that I'm in. Skin equality across all industries and professions is the goal - let's do this!

C. R. Cooper

The Skin Theologian

IG: @theskintheologian

DON'T DO IT! 3 REASONS WHY POPPING THAT PIMPLE IS THE LAST THING YOU WANT TO DO!

Don't forget
Go to www.skintheologian.com for your FREE gift.

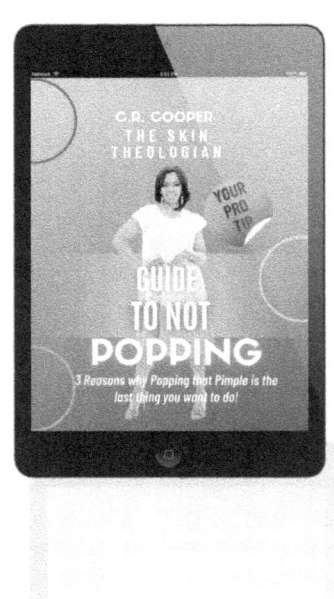

SKIN COLOR IN DERMATOLOGY TEXTBOOKS: AN UPDATED EVALUATION AND ANALYSIS

Benefits of Melanin

How False Beliefs in Physical Medical Differences Still Lives On

OUR SCIENCE, HER MAGIC

Dermatology has a problem with skin color

How we fail black patients in pain

Why doesn't everybody have dark skin today?

World's oldest fossils found in Morocco

Humans did not stem from one ancestor

Women of color spend more than $8 billion on bleaching creams worldwide every year

www.ingramcontent.com/pod-product-compliance
Lightning Source LLC
Chambersburg PA
CBHW020258030426
42336CB00010B/832